Cheickna Konaté

Studies of candidiasis in infants

Cheickna Konaté

Studies of candidiasis in infants

using diapers at the Mali hospital

ScienciaScripts

Cover image: www.ingimage.com

This book is a translation from the original published under ISBN 978-620-6-71648-8.

Publisher:
Sciencia Scripts
is a trademark of
Dodo Books Indian Ocean Ltd. and OmniScriptum S.R.L publishing group

120 High Road, East Finchley, London, N2 9ED, United Kingdom
Str. Armeneasca 28/1, office 1, Chisinau MD-2012, Republic of Moldova, Europe
Printed at: see last page
ISBN: 978-620-5-48226-1

DEDICATION

DEDICATION

I dedicate this work :

- To my father Youssouf KONATE
- To mother Alima COULIBALY
- To my wife Alima DIARRA
- To my daughter Halimatou KONATE
- To my son Cheick Abdoul Kader KONATE

Dad, Mom, thank you.

ACKNOWLEDGEMENTS

ACKNOWLEDGEMENTS

I thank the Merciful, the Most Merciful, the Builder of builders, the Builder of the heavens and the earth and his prophet MOHAMED peace and salvation upon him.

My thanks to :

- My big brothers
- My big sisters
- The KONATE family and the COULIBALY family
- My friends and the entire 1[ière] class of the Master in Medical Biology Engineering
- My teachers from registration to today

I would like to express my sincere thanks to all the staff at Mali Hospital in general, and to the Laboratory and Pediatrics staff in particular, for their warm welcome.

I would like to extend my warmest thanks to all those who have contributed in any way to our supervision.

CONTENTS

TABLE OF CONTENTS

INTRODUCTION

I. Introduction

Candidiasis or moniliasis are cosmopolitan diseases caused by ***ubiquitous Candida*** yeasts, frequently isolated from the environment (air, soil, fruit, food products, dairy products, cereals). In humans, they colonize numerous sites and live commensally in the digestive, upper air and genitourinary mucosa, as well as on the skin surface [1]. ***Candida***, formerly known as ***Monilia***, are at the limit of perfect and imperfect dimorphism. By virtue of their teleomorphic sexual reproduction, they belong to the phylum Ascomycotinae. Through anamorphic asexual reproduction, the *Candida* genus belongs to the Deuteromycotinae division [2]. They are unicellular fungal elements called blastospores because their budding is of the blastic type, measuring 3 to 6 µm in diameter, round to oval, budding or not and producing or not a pseudo filament (false filament) or a true filament [2]. In the actual infection or candidiasis, the yeast multiplies, taking on its filamentous form (pseudomycelium) and becoming pathogenic. *Candida* yeasts are responsible for over 80% of yeast infections in humans, and *Candida albicans* is implicated in 90% of cases. Frequently encountered in the immunocompromised, the elderly and infants. Diaper dermatitis is a frequent complaint in infants [2]. Irritant or convex dermatitis is an erythematous dermatitis that starts at the diaper rubbing areas, reaching the buttocks, external genitalia and thighs, forming a W shape and respecting the folds. In most cases, breech dermatitis is linked to mechanical factors, with occlusion and maceration playing an initiating role. Convex or "W-shaped" dermatitis is the most frequently encountered breech dermatitis. Peak incidence occurs between 6 and 12 months of age. It is multifactorial in origin, linked to the characteristics of the infant's skin and to perineo-gluteal occlusion [3]. Because of infant incontinence, the diaper area is constantly under attack from more or less corrosive urine or feces. The alkalinity of the urinary pH, increased by fecal bacterial ureases, bile salts, proteases and lipases, all contribute to skin aggression. Yeasts present in stools can cause superinfection. In infants, diaper rash can develop very rapidly, particularly in the event of diarrhea [4]. In some cases, the perianal area is directly affected, due to chemical irritation in the event of diarrhoea, which runs counter to the strict "W" pattern. Fold bottoms are respected, but may be secondarily affected in cases of massive ***Candida*** colonization. These different manifestations are very different from congenital cutaneous candidiasis of newborns, linked to genital candidiasis, which is an infection of women during genital activity; and also from nosocomial candidiasis, and the use of other ropes or traditional protective objects commonly known as "Tiélabagani", which end up irritating the skin [2]. These clinical manifestations can slow down an infant's psychomotor development as a result of negligence or even incomplete treatment, and could have far more serious consequences, especially in young girls, such as sterility or infertility. The goal of zero candidiasis through diaper use in infants is possible. Numerous studies on preventive measures and effective management are already available. Including these different aspects in a health education policy and necessarily in the ongoing training of health workers could contribute considerably to reducing health concerns linked to the use of diapers in infants. The diaper normally used to help parents ultimately harms the infant's health. Candidiasis linked to diaper use, and especially to the use of second-hand diapers, is essentially behavioral in nature, due to the attention paid to diaper changing. Socially and culturally constructed relationships in reference to the behavior, activities and attributes of women in our society, particularly those activities that take place mainly within the family, could influence diapering. Socio-economic reasons that are sometimes difficult to explain lead to the undesirable use of diapers, with diapers changing at least every 7 hours, sometimes incomprehensible that a diaper can last longer. However, these clinical manifestations are much less frequent in families who have difficulty even obtaining a diaper for reasons of poverty. Laziness to change diapers properly, or ignorance of the consequences of inappropriate diaper use, add to this the relevant cosmopolitan nature of ***Candida*** [5].

Given the evolution of our societies, it is necessary to take into account certain sanitary and hygienic aspects, especially for our little ones, in order to respond more adequately to society's needs.

Today, communication for behavior change is necessary, and pediatric services are overwhelmed by the issue, hence the interest of this study.

OBJECTIVES

Objectives

- ✓ **General objective**

Study candidiasis in infants using diapers.

- ✓ **Specific objectives**

1. Describe the clinical signs of candidal diaper rash in infants
2. Identify risk factors for candidiasis associated with diaper rash in infants.
3. Describe the role of the mycology laboratory in the diagnosis and prevention of cutaneous candidiasis in infants.

GENERAL

II. General

A. Clinical signs of diaper rash [10].

According to L.FERTITTA, the diagnostic approach to diaper rash should involve analysis of the following elements:

- Seat location: convexities, folds, diffuse
- Elementary lesions: pustules, vesicles, papules, erosions, ulcerations, scales.
- Associated functional signs: pruritus, sleep disorders, pain.
- The presence of distant skin lesions: scalp, other folds, extremities.
- The presence of general signs: fever, decline or break in saturo-ponderal growth, eating disorders.
- Background and history :
  - personal and family history, including dermatological: psoriasis, atopy, digestive disease responsible for diarrhoea;
  - treatments: topicals applied, especially for diaper changes, oral treatments administered, type of diapers, etc. ;
  - evolution: acute or chronic nature of the rash, presence of flare-ups, their frequency and duration, factors triggering or calming flare-ups

Irritant dermatitis of the convexities is also known as "W" erythema: the lesions form a "W" shape when the child is examined supine, with legs raised. In the most severe forms, the lesions may spread to the entire seat, but also in cases of superinfection, particularly with *Candida*. Macules and papules are most common, but a rapidly spreading, vesicular or even erosive form also exists. Involvement is well limited. Its pathophysiology is usually multifactorial, combining physical factors (diaper occlusion, maceration, friction), chemical factors (alkaline urinary pH, bacterial fecal ureases, bile salts, etc.) and microbiological factors (superinfections by commensal bacteria and yeasts of the skin and digestive tract). All these factors contribute to maceration at the seat-layer interface, which explains its location on the convexities.

Candidiasis in infants due to diaper use must be distinguished from :

- psoriasis of diapers: the main differential diagnosis for irritant dermatitis is psoriasis of diapers, which also tends to be located on the convexities, although it may later spread to the folds. When it is diffuse, it often extends to the roots of the thighs. Analysis of the elementary lesions enables us to differentiate it from "classic" W erythema.
- Contact dermatitis of immuno-allergic origin is rare and frequently mistaken for irritant dermatitis. Clinically, it is a contact eczema associating erythematous, vesicular, oozing and sometimes crusty lesions.
- Infant seborrheic dermatitis, due to colonization with yeasts of the Malassezia genus, predominates in the folds. It can also spread to the whole seat. There is frequently bipolar involvement of seborrheic areas (scalp and face).
- *Candida* intertrigo, in particular *Candida albicans*, is both a frequent cause of diaper rash and an all-too-frequent cause of diaper rash.
- Infant scabies may have a preferred topography in the folds (inguinal, gluteal, axillary).
- Perivulvar erythema and vulvitis can occur in the context of higher urinary or gynecological infections.

These different manifestations are quite different from congenital cutaneous candidiasis of the newborn, linked to genital candidiasis, which is an infection of women during periods of genital activity. This is a frequent reason for consultation in gynecology, and can affect 8.8% to 63% of women; and also nosocomial candidiasis and the use of other ropes or traditional protective objects commonly known as Tiélabagani, which end up irritating the skin.

Other clinical aspects need to be taken into account in management

- Zinc deficiency should also be suspected when erythematous and erosive lesions predominate in the periorificial areas, rapidly spreading to the entire seat.
- Kawasaki disease should be suspected in the presence of diaper rash associated with prolonged fever lasting more than 5 days and other major clinical or biological criteria of the disease: adenopathy, cheilitis, edematous erythema of the extremities.
- A primary immune deficiency should also be considered in the presence of diffuse, atypical diaper rash, especially when associated with other cutaneous and/or infectious manifestations.

- ❖ Rules for applying cosmetics must be adapted to the child's age, especially in the case of newborns whose skin is more permeable. In general, all irritating substances that may cause sensitization should be avoided (certain perfumes or natural essential oils such as orange blossom, bergamot, lemon, etc.).

Taking into account all the preliminary information provided by parents on the history of diaper rash in infants, its evolution, the presence or absence of elementary ulceration lesions, associated functional signs of pain, the presence of skin lesions at a distance from the scalp or other folds, the presence of general signs of fever, and treatment, particularly in traditional medicine with plant- or plant-part-based decocts. Infant diaper rash is a diaper dermatitis caused by skin irritation. It is characterized by dry or oozing redness, with or without small pimples. In the most severe cases, the skin may be raw, accompanied by burning sensations, cracks or ulcerations. It generally appears on areas in contact with the diaper. It takes the form of a W covering the inner thighs, buttocks and pubis. When soaked with urine, the erythema spreads to the lower back and abdomen, and into the skin folds of the infant's thighs and buttocks. When stools are acidic (diarrhea), erythema appears around the anus and spreads rapidly.

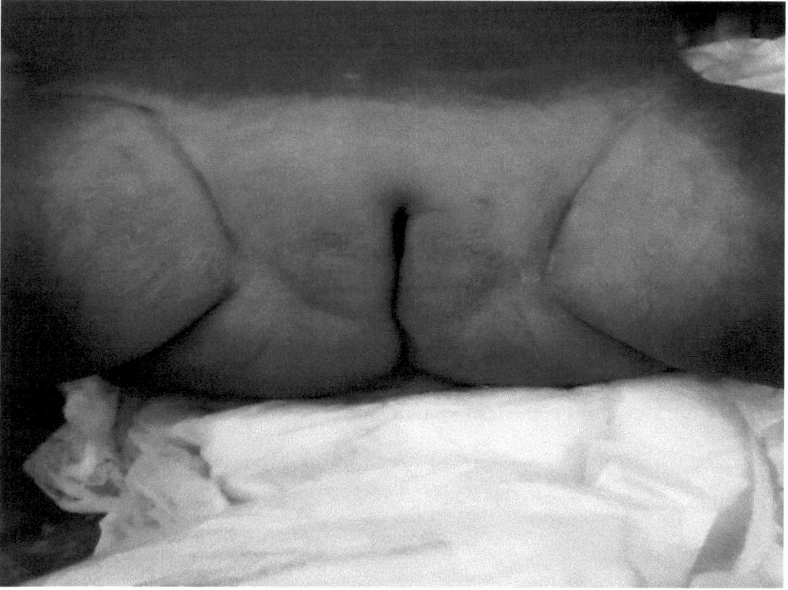

Figure 1: Candidiasis diaper rash in infants.

Source: Mali Hospital Pediatrics Department

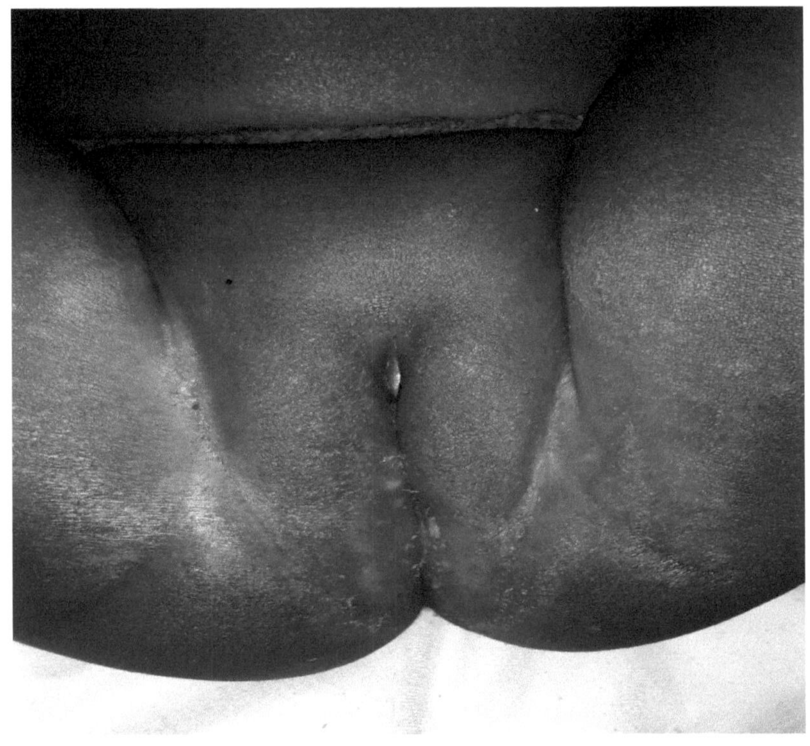

Figure 2: Candidiasis diaper rash in infants.

Source: Mali Hospital Pediatrics Department

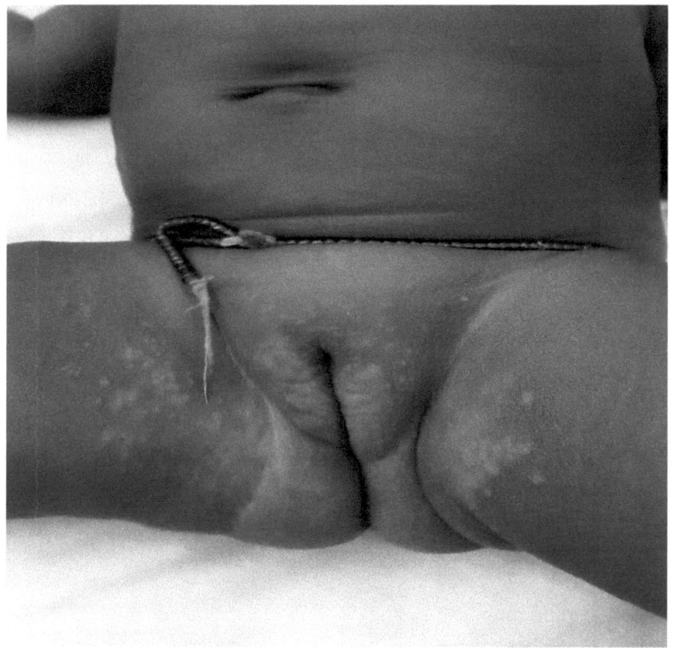

Figure 3: Candidiasis diaper rash in infants.

Source: Mali Hospital Pediatrics Department

B. **Biological diagnosis [2]**

Mycological diagnosis comprises 4 important stages:

- sampling,
- direct examination,
- culture on appropriate media,
- and identification of the isolated fungus. A study of sensitivity to antifungal agents can be carried out if required.

1. **Withdrawal**

Rub lesions with 2 sterile swabs moistened with sterile distilled water (one for direct examination, the other for culture).

Sampling is an important step. The reliability of a mycological examination depends largely on the quality of the sample.

Samples should be taken at a distance from any antifungal therapy, and sent rapidly to the laboratory for immediate inoculation, to avoid the risk of false-negative results due to desiccation (especially in the case of moist samples such as swabs), which is often detrimental to yeast viability, and to avoid invasion by saprophytic flora.

For dry skin lesions, scrape the scales from the periphery with vaccinostyl or a scalpel blade and place in sterile petri dishes. Squeeze erythematous irritant breech dermatitis and swab for serosities.

For mucous lesions, whitish coatings are swabbed with a sterile swab. Swabbing is also performed for peri-anal lesions. In the case of sepsis, blood is taken under rigorous aseptic conditions: 1 to 3 ml of blood for blood culture, which is not really recommended for superficial candidiasis, particularly in the case of candidiasis linked to irritant diaper dermatitis in infants.

2. Direct examination

This direct examination, an essential technique for revealing the fungus in a "parasitic state", provides formal proof of mycosis in just a few minutes. Direct examination of the sample enables rapid orientation of the diagnosis. Its quality depends on the quality of the sample, which must be taken by competent personnel. Fresh" direct examination is performed directly on the swab slide, without fixation or specific staining. It is facilitated by the use of brighteners (notably Lugol's). *Candida* blastospores, possibly accompanied by pseudomycelium, can be detected.

For direct examination of slides after staining, the usual stains are available, notably Methylene Blue, May Grunwald Giemsa and, above all, Gram stain.

In addition, Indian ink staining enables differential diagnosis of encapsulated yeast, notably *cryptococcus neoformans* of the *candida* genus.

3. Culture

Isolated yeasts can grow on the classic culture media used in microbiology (ordinary agar, blood agar, heart-brain broth....). Sabouraud's medium is the most suitable, however, and Petri dishes offer a larger plating surface than tubes.On the other hand, there is a risk of contamination by airborne mold spores through inoculation and handling of the dishes, but they enable good isolation of colonies and visualization of yeast associations.

Standard media, especially Sabouraud agar media with added chloramphenicol and/or gentamycin, are the most widely used. Cycloheximide (actidione®), often associated with these media, can inhibit the growth of many molds likely to contaminate cultures; ideal for *Candida albicans,* they can also inhibit or slow down the growth of yeasts of the *Candida* genus such as *Candida glabrata*, *Candida parapsilosis*, *Candida tropicalis* and *Candida famata*.

Growth temperature depends on the sampling site. For superficial samples, plates are incubated between 25°C-27°C. For deep samples, cultures are incubated at 37°C. An incubation period of 24 to 48 hours is sufficient to isolate the majority of pathogenic yeasts belonging to the *Candida* genus.

Chromogenic media: these media, to which chromogenic substances are added, impart a particular coloration to the colonies growing on them, which varies according to the species. In most cases, this coloration is based on the detection of hexosaminidase-type enzymatic activity (N-acetyl-α-D-galactosaminidase). Bacterial multiplication is also inhibited. More expensive than traditional Sabouraud media, these media nevertheless save 24 to 48 hours, since yeasts can be identified in many cases immediately after isolation and without subsequent subculturing, given the high prevalence of the species concerned. They are also particularly interesting for sites likely to host several species, notably in monitoring the colonization of patients at risk of developing superficial candidiasis in the breech area through the use of diapers in infants, since they enable yeast associations to be visualized directly.

Fluorogenic media, such as Fluoroplate Candida (Merck), enable the growth of *Candida albicans* colonies in 24 to 48 h of incubation, which show a bluish fluorescence when the plates are observed under ultraviolet light (366 nm). The need for specific equipment limits the use of this medium.

4. Identification

Identification tests can only be carried out in the presence of well-individualized colonies. In current practice, identification of the various *Candida* species is based on morphological, physiological and, more recently, immunological characteristics, using tests based on agglutination of latex particles sensitized with monoclonal antibodies. Mass spectrometry and molecular biology, although promising, are currently only available to specialized centers and research teams. Since *Candida albicans is* the species most frequently isolated and considered the most virulent, the first step in the diagnostic process is to identify it. A number of tests have therefore been developed, with varying degrees of rapidity and specifically adapted to its identification. These include the blastesis (or germination) test, performed by incubating the isolate for 2 to 4 hours on rabbit plasma at 35-37°C, and the chlamydosporulation test, based on sub-culturing the isolate for 24 to 48 hours at 25-28°C in deep streaks in PCB (potato, carrot, bile) or RAT (rice, agar, tween 80) *Candida albicans* is then identified respectively by the production of a thin germ tube of homogeneous diameter without constriction at its base emerging from the mother cell or by the production of chlamydospores, rounded structures 10 to 15 µm in diameter with a thick wall (double contour appearance) produced singly or in clusters at the tip of the pseudomycelium.

Numerous parameters (observer experience, inoculum load, pH, etc.) that can affect the result of the blastesis test, and the risk associated with plasma handling, have led to the gradual abandonment of this test. At the same time, the time required to obtain the results of the chlamydosporulation test is reducing its use. In addition, these two tests are unable to differentiate *Candida dubliniensis from Candida albicans*, and have been replaced by faster and/or more specific tests.

Biochemical **tests**

When colonies on chromogenic media fail to give a characteristic coloration, and rapid tests prove negative, a wide range of identification strips can be used routinely. These are essential for identifying species other than *Candida albicans*. These tests are mainly based on reactions involving the assimilation of carbohydrates under aerobic conditions (auxanogram) or their fermentation under anaerobic conditions (zymogram). Chromogenic substrate hydrolysis, enzyme detection and cycloheximide resistance can also be studied in conjunction with these assimilation tests. Depending on the systems on the market, these reactions are reflected in the appearance of a cloudy cup or a pH indicator turn. The profile obtained, translated into numerical code, is then compared with databases enabling the identification of up to 63 species (ID®32C gallery) of yeast, depending on the system. A fully automated phenotypic identification system, the Vitek 2, offers reduced handling time and rapid identification results (18 h).

AUXACOLOR™2 is the biochemical auxanogram identification test used at the Mali Hospital Laboratory Department. The AUXACOLOR™2 gallery identifies 31 yeast species. 92.5% of strains tested are identified within 48h (59.2% within 24h). The AUXACOLOR™2 gallery differentiates all *Candida dubliniensis* (5 strains tested) and *Candida albicans* (15 strains) strains.

CandiSelect™4 or PCB culture carried out in parallel with AUXACOLOR™2 testing, enables yeast associations to be visualized.

Yeast identification is based on both biochemical characteristics, determined using microplates, and morphological characteristics, preferably determined on PCB or RAT medium. All these data are essential for a complete identification.

In addition, the origin of the samples and the clinical context of candidiasis in infants through the use of diapers were taken into account when interpreting the results.

Immunological methods :

These tests are based on the principle of agglutination of latex particles sensitized with monoclonal antibodies specifically recognizing a wall antigen of the different species. Bichro-latex®albicans (Fumouze Diagnostics) identifies the *Candida albicans* / *Candida dubliniensis* complex.

Enzymatic methods

The fungiscreen® test (Bio-rad) takes the form of a mini-gallery with 6 cups and studies 7 characteristics. Detection of 5 specific enzymes, Tetrazolium reduction and Trehalose assimilation are indicated by a color change.

In fact, the diagnosis of candidiasis linked to diaper-related irritant breech dermatitis in infants is based on a comparison of clinical and paraclinical data. Culture results must be treated critically, given the saprophytic and cosmopolitan nature of the *Candida* genus. Quantifying colonies on culture can help in the therapeutic decision.

C. Therapeutics [2]

Superficial candidiasis, particularly in cases of candidiasis linked to irritant diaper dermatitis in infants; cutaneous galenic forms are in greater demand. The therapeutic objective is to destroy the pathogen, cure the patient and avoid complications.

After use of bicarbonate solutions or soaps, aqueous antiseptics (iodine derivatives, chlorhexidine); ointments, creams or lotions for twice-daily local application, and increasingly popular spray forms. Treatment continues until cured. For prevention, apply oxyplastine cream to the diaper area before wearing a diaper.

The mechanism of action of the main antifungal agents is an action on membrane ergosterol or its synthesis.

POLYENES

1. Amphotericin B

Amphotericin B is an antifungal agent for both yeast-forming and filamentous fungal pathogens, and the standard treatment for severe mycoses. Isolated in 1955 from *Streptomyces nodosus*, polyene forms insoluble complexes with *Candida* membrane sterols, altering cell permeability. Oral absorption is very low, does not cross the intestinal barrier and is non-toxic. Intravenous administration produces a sufficiently high blood concentration, with high toxicity and immediate reactions upon first prescription: chills, fever, general malaise, digestive disorders, and secondary reactions of renal toxicity, notably moderate urea elevation and irreversible toxic nephropathy.

Amphotericin B in 100mg/ml oral suspension, 50mg powder for injection. Dosage is 50 mg/kg/day for infants and children (1 measuring pipette for 2 kg/day), four times a day after meals, until symptoms disappear. Dermal forms for twice-daily local application are also available.

2. Nystatin

Discovered in 1950, extracted from the mycelium of *Streptomyces noursei*, polyene. The mechanism of action is based on the binding of nystatin to sterols (ergosterol). The spectrum of action is limited to yeasts. Digestive absorption is nil; orally, 32% of the administered dose is found unchanged in the feces. The absence of an injectable form is due to poor tolerance. Oral and local routes are very well tolerated, with low toxicity. Dosage for infants is 5 to 30 ml per day (i.e. 500,000 to 3 million IU) and for children:

10 to 40 ml per day (i.e. 1 to 4 million IU). Dermal forms are available as twice-daily local applications.

IMIDAZOLE DERIVATIVES

1. Miconazole

Imidazoles inhibit ergosterol biosynthesis in fungal membranes. Broad spectrum of action against yeasts and certain filamentous fungi. Per os some nausea and vomiting, intravenous not nephrotoxic. Avoid association with Amphotericin **B.** Local twice-daily skin applications are available.

2. Ketoconazole

Active against yeasts (*candida, Malassezia*) and dermatophytes. Good tissue penetration, particularly in sebaceous glands. Concentration in CSF is low. Excretion is mainly faecal. Cytolytic liver toxicity regresses on discontinuation of the drug. A transaminase assay is therefore required prior to treatment, and fortnightly monitoring should be instituted in the event of prolonged use. The daily dose for children is 7 mg/kg *per os*. Dermal forms for twice-daily local application are available

3. TRIAZOLES

The azole nucleus contains 3 nitrogen atoms. Fluconazole diffuses well into CSF and saliva, and is eliminated in the urine in its active form. Active against *candida and cryptococcus* yeasts. Itraconazole has good tissue concentration in the lung, kidney and brain, and limited toxicity, but liver monitoring is necessary. Cutaneous forms are available as twice-daily local applications

FLUCYTOSINE

5-Fluorocytosine (5FC) is a fluorinated pyrimidine synthesized in 1957, mainly active against yeast fungi. Prohibited as monotherapy due to the emergence of resistant mutants in yeast infections. Very good distribution throughout the body, particularly in the CSF. In cases of renal insufficiency, FLUCYTOSINE accumulates in plasma, causing nausea and vomiting when taken orally; severe hematological accidents (aplasia, agranulocytosis) have only been described in immunocompromised patients (AIDS) or those with severe renal insufficiency.

D. Traditional Medicine

Moreover, not in the context of modern traditional medicine based on studies in pharmaceutical science, in particular pharmacognosy, but rather in the context of traditional African and Malian medicine, which generally involves mothers of infants intuitively consulting or seeking advice on the preparation of one or more plant-based recipes or parts of plants (roots, bark, stems and leaves) as a decoction for the treatment of Candidiasis in infants through the use of diapers.

Table I: List of plants traditionally used for the treatment of Candidiasis in infants through the use of diapers.

N°	Scientific name of plant	Common name (in Bambara) of the plant	Plant or plant part used
1	***Parkia biglobosa***	Néré	Bark
2	***Acacia Senegalensis***	Patougou	Bark
3	***Butosperma paradoxum or Vitellaria paradoxa***	Shea	Bark
4	***Sclerocarya birrea***	Gouna	Bark
5	***Eclipta prostrata***	Moussofi	Racine
6	***Acacia nilotica***	Boina	Seed
7	***Sygzygium aromaticum*** (The clove tree)	Bénéfoutou	Flower buds (cloves)
8	***Acacia occidentalis***	Soumafaga	Bark
9	***Stylosantes ercta or mucronata***	djofaga or somafaga	Whole plant

The decoction recipe is generally composed of nine plants. Combinations of three or four herbs may be used, depending on the locality.

METHODOLOGY

III. Methodology

1. Study setting and location

Our study was carried out in the Pediatrics Department and the Laboratory Department of Mali Hospital, where pediatric consultations and routine biological and mycological examinations are carried out at the request of prescribers.

Hôpital du Mali is a public hospital, the fruit of SinoMalian cooperation. Hôpital du Mali was created by law N^{0} 10-010 of May 20, 2010 and inaugurated on September 23, 2010. Hôpital du Mali is located at the southern exit of the 3ème bridge in the city of Bamako, a few meters from the banks of the Niger River.

The Mali Hospital's main missions are :

- Diagnosis, treatment and follow-up of patients
- Handling emergencies and referrals
- Participate in the initial and continuing training of healthcare professionals
- Conduct research in the medical field.

2. Type and duration of study

This is a 10-month prospective descriptive study from July 2020 to April 2021.

3. Study population

All infant patients seen in the pediatric department with diaper-related breech dermatitis during the study period.

4. Inclusion criteria

We included all infants with diaper dermatitis.

5. Non-inclusion criteria: Patients who did not meet the inclusion criteria.

6. Ethical aspects :

- Authorization from Mali Hospital management
- Free and informed consent of parents
- Declaration of conflict of interest
- The anonymity and confidentiality of the files were respected.

7. Study parameters

- Age
- The sex

- Mother's occupation
- Place of residence
- Mother's family situation
- Mother's level of education
- Clinical signs of diaper rash candidiasis
- *Candida albicans* candidiasis
- Diaper marks in infants

8. Laboratory techniques

The technique used for biological and mycological diagnosis is manual.

Withdrawal

- Sterile swab: STERILE EO
- Saline solution: 0.9% saline injection/500ml
- Sterile syringe: 10ml.

Identification of sample taken :

- Name and surname
- Order number
- The date

Local organization of mycological diagnostics

At Mali Hospital's laboratory department, mycological diagnosis is carried out in the large bacteriology room, where we have all the necessary equipment.

Materials and reagents used

- Blades and slats
- Saline solution
- Disposable plastic handle
- Gram staining reagent kit
- Sabouraud culture medium
- Refrigerators
- PSM (Microbiological Safety Station): Raecho International MODEL : RBSC
- Oven: incubator RPPH-140A

- Optical microscope: OPTIKA B-383PLi
- AUXACOLOR™2 gallery

Biological diagnostic procedure

- **Swab sampling**

The swab is applied to the irritation or even the lesion, and closed pus can be gently squeezed.

- **Inoculation on ordinary Sabouraud culture medium**

After inoculation on ordinary Sabouraud culture medium in petri dishes and incubation or culture within 24 to 48 hours, whitish colonies of more or less regular size and outline and more or less uniform yellowish colonies of one or more types generally below the whitish colonies characteristic of the presence of yeast on Sabouraud medium.

Macroscopic observation of yeast colonies of the *Candida* genus on Sabouraud medium, while appreciating color, odor and size, gives a characteristic idea of the species identified. Subculturing on Sabouraud medium is sometimes necessary for isolation and to facilitate various identification tests.

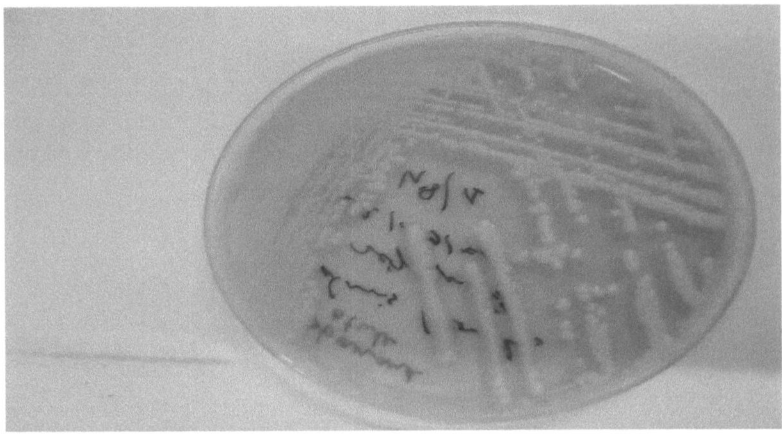

Figure 1: Isolated colonies of *Candida* yeast on Sabouraud medium.

Source: Mali Hospital laboratory department.

- **Fresh state**

The fresh state is a prerequisite for culture. After cultivation on Sabouraud medium, a whitish colony is placed on a slide mixed with physiological water and covered with a coverslip, then observed under a microscope with a 10* then 40* objective. The presence of a yeast spore is characteristic, with or without budding, and sometimes with the presence of pseudomycelium, mycelium or even chlamydospore.

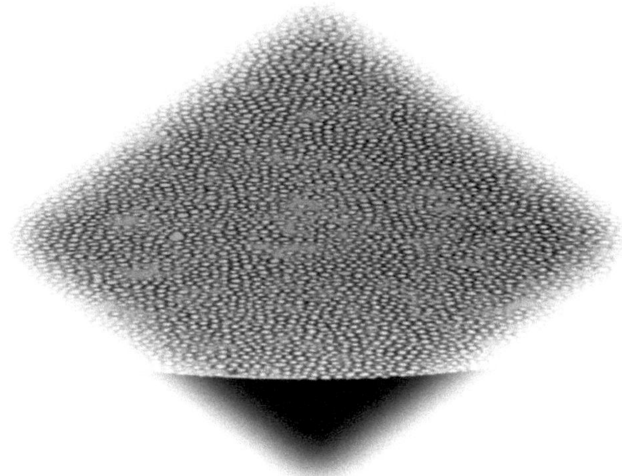

Figure 2: *Candida* yeasts observed in the fresh state.

Source: Mali Hospital laboratory department.

- **Gram staining**

After spreading the whitish colony on Sabouraud culture medium. The slide is air-dried then heat-fixed, and after cooling, the Gram staining technique is applied. Yeasts are most clearly visible in Gram-positive violet impregnation.

Yellowish or other colonies on Sabouraud culture medium after spreading on a slide and using the Gram staining technique, various bacteria can be observed, in particular gram-positive cocci and gram-negative bacilli, certainly testifying to contamination or superinfection related to fecal flora in the infant's breech area.

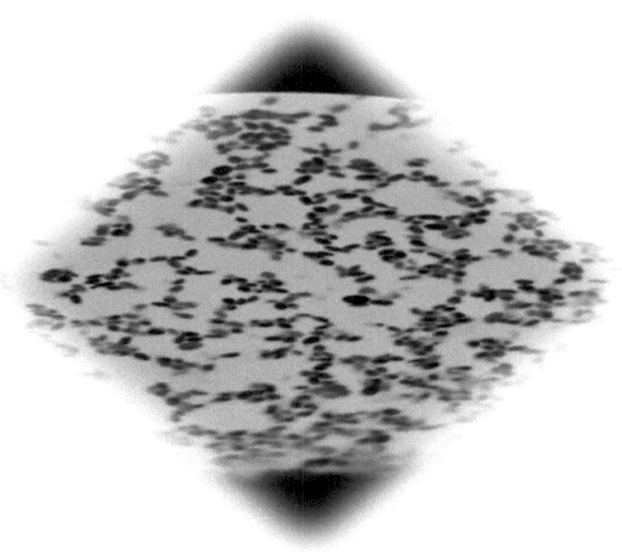

Figure 3: *Candida* yeasts observed after Gram staining.

Source: Mali Hospital laboratory department.

- **Blastèse test**

Search for filamentation on serum at 37°c (detection of *candida albicans*)

In a sterile stoppered hemolysis tube:

Emulsify a white porcelain colony isolated on Sabouraud medium in 1 ml serum (patient of the day).

Incubate 3 hours at 37°C

After 3 hours, observe a drop of the suspension under the microscope and note the filamentation of the yeasts.

Positive filamentation: *Candida albicans*

Negative filamentation: other *Candida* or yeast species

- **Identification using the Auxacolor2 test**

The AUXACOLOR™2 gallery is an identification system whose principle is based on the assimilation of sugars. Yeast growth is visualized by turning a pH indicator.

After subculturing the inoculum prepared from a 24 to 48-hour culture on Sabouraud medium. Under sterile conditions, inoculate the suspension medium (R2) with colonies of pure strain in sufficient quantity (1 to 5 identical colonies) to obtain an opacity equal to 1.5 McFarland. It is necessary to respect the opacity of the inoculum to guarantee the quality of the results. Homogenize the suspension using a vortex. Pipette 100µl of inoculum into each well of the microplate (R1). Cover the microplate (R1) with the adhesive, ensuring perfectly uniform adhesion. Incubate 48h (72h if necessary) at 37° C.

The 16 biochemical characteristics, divided into 15 cups (POX and PRO tests are combined in the same cup), are used for identification.

A 5-digit numerical profile is obtained by grouping by 3 the values of the 15 biochemical tests, and this is searched in a database for species identification.

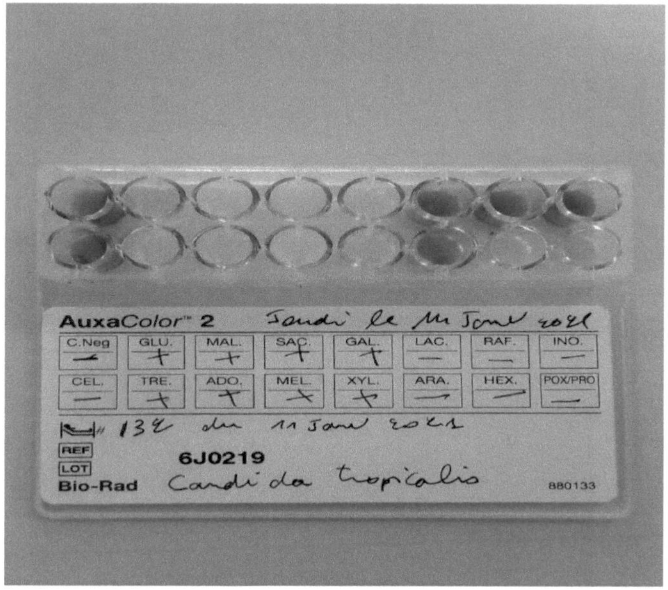

Figure 4: ***Candida tropicalis*** **species identified.**

Source: Mali Hospital laboratory department.

RESULTS

IV. Results

1. Overall results

Our study included 161 infants with diaper dermatitis whose clinical diagnosis and tests were carried out respectively in the Pediatrics Department and the Laboratory Department of Mali Hospital.

The 0-12 months age group was the most represented with 86.33%. The sex ratio was 1.09, i.e. 109 boys for every 100 girls. Bulk thrift store diapers were by far the most widely used, at 74.52%. The majority of samples tested, 47.5%, were identified as *Candida albicans.*

The majority of infant mothers were married. Patients residing in the commune VI of Bamako were more represented.

2. Socio-demographic results

Table I: Distribution of infants according to age

Age (Months)	Workforce	Percentage
0-6	89	55,28
6-12	50	31,05
12-18	9	5,6
18-24	11	6,83
>24	2	1,24
Total	161	100

55, 28% of infants were less than or equal to 6 months old.

31.05% of infants were aged between 6 and 12 months.

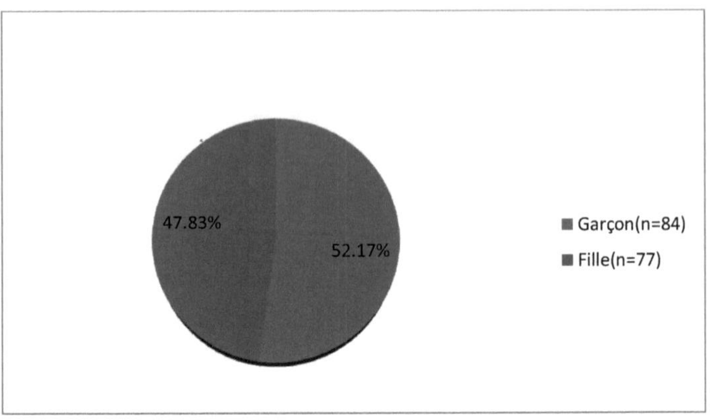

Figure 5: Distribution of infants by sex

Boys were slightly in the majority, with a sex ratio of 1.09.

Table II: Distribution of infants by place of residence

Place of residence	Workforce	Percentage
Commune VI	141	87,6
Commune V	4	2,48
Commune III	1	0,62
Commune II	2	1,24
Commune I	5	3,1
Kati	8	4,96
Total	161	100

Patients residing in Commune VI were more represented, at 87.6%.

Table III: Distribution of infants according to mother's occupation

Mother's occupation	Workforce	Percentage

Housekeeper	88	54,7
Retailer	24	14,9
Student	10	6,2
Student	9	5,6
Health agents	6	3,72
Artisane	6	3,72
Secretary	5	3,1
Uniform wearer	5	3,1
Accountant	3	1,86
Teacher	2	1,24
Animator	2	1,24
Legal	1	0,62
Total	161	100

The most represented socio-professional stratum was housewives with 54.7%, followed by shopkeepers with 14.9%.

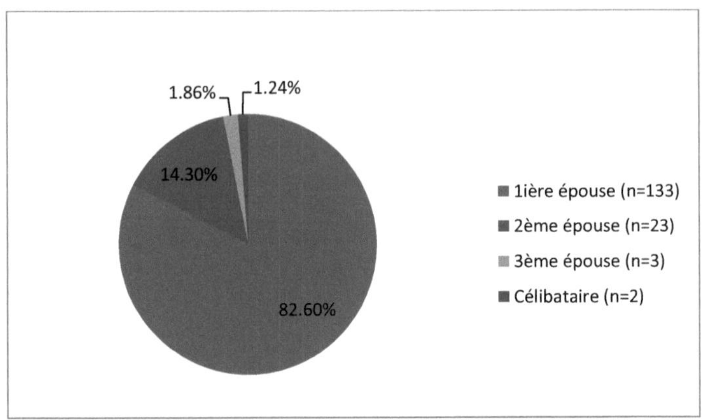

Figure 6: Distribution of infants according to mother's marital status.

In the study population, 98.76% of mothers of infants were married, 82.60% of whom were first wives, followed by second wives (14.30%).

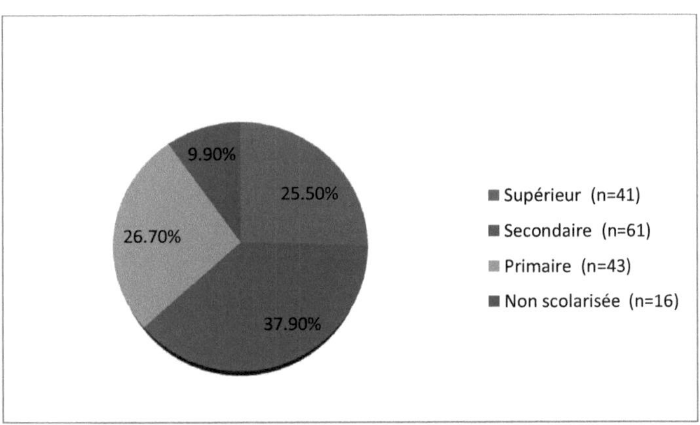

Figure 7: Distribution of infants by mother's level of education

The majority of mothers of infants, 90.1%, had attended school, with secondary education at 37.9%, followed by primary education at 26.7% and higher education at 25.5%.

Table IV: Distribution of infants according to diaper brand

Coat mark	Workforce	Percentage
Fripes-en vrac	120	74,52
Non Fripes	41	25,48
Total	161	100

Bulk thrift store diapers, 74.52%, were by far the most used, followed by Non Fripes diapers at 25.48%.

3. Mycological results

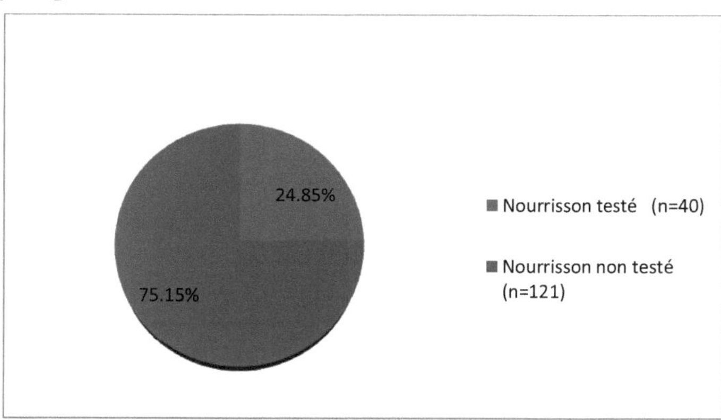

Figure 8: Distribution of infants according to test

24.85% of samples were taken and tested.

Table V: Distribution of infants tested according to fungus isolated

Mushrooms	Workforce	Percentage
Candida albicans	19	47,5
Candida lipolytica	9	22,5
Candida dubliniensis	4	10
Candida zeylanoides	4	10
Candida parapsilosis	2	5

Candida tropicalis	2	5
Total	40	100

Of the samples tested, 47.5% were identified as *Candida albicans*, followed by *Candida lipolytica* (22.5%).

10% were identified as *Candida dubliniensis* and *Candida zeylanoides* respectively.

5% were identified for each of the species *Candida parapsilosis* and *Candida tropicalis.*

Table VI: Layer distribution by isolated fungus

Coating marks	Isolated mushrooms												total
	Candida albicans		*Candida lipolytica*		*Candida dubliniensis*		*Candida zeylanoides*		*Candida parapsilosis*		*Candida tropicalis*		
	No.	*%*	*No.*	*%*	*No*	*%*	*No.*	*%*	*No.*	*%*	*No.*	*%*	
Fripes-en Vrac	13	65	9	100	3	75	4	100	1	50	1	50	30
Non Fripes	6	35	0	0	1	25	0	0	1	50	1	50	10
Total	19	100	9	100	4	100	4	100	2	100	2	100	40

Of the *candida albicans* isolated, 65% were in infants using bulk cloth diapers and 20% in those using the Sewa brand.

100% of the *candida lipolytica* isolated were from infants using bulk cloth diapers.

Of the *candida dubliniensis* isolated, 75% were in infants using bulk cloth diapers.

100% of the *candida zeylanoides* isolated were in infants using bulk cloth diapers.

The proportion of candidiasis in infants per diaper use differed significantly between bulk Fripes and Non Fripes diapers ($p<0.01$).

COMMENTS AND DISCUSSION

V. Comments and discussion

1. Demographics

Of the 161 infants included in our study, 55.28% were less than or equal to 6 months of age (≤ 6 months), 31.05% between 6-12 months, 5.6% between 12-18 months, 6.83% between 18-24 months and 1.24% over 24 months (> 24 months). Dominique Tennstedt finds that the peak incidence is essentially between 6 and 12 months. There may also be a peak during the first 4 weeks of life (probably due to liquid stools associated with breastfeeding) [13].

Girls accounted for 47.83% and boys for a slight majority at 52.17%. La *Revue Médicale de Liège 2006;* Infants' breech skin is subjected to numerous aggressions, largely conditioned by the wearing of diapers. The condition, of an acute inflammatory nature, is common and affects girls and boys with equal frequency. It is most prevalent in babies aged between 7 and 15 months [17].

Among mothers of infants, the most represented socio-professional stratum was housewives with 54.7%, followed by shopkeepers with 14.9%. In the study population, 98.76% of infant mothers were married, 82.60% of them first wives, followed by second wives at 14.30%. The majority of mothers, 90.1%, had attended school, with secondary education at 37.9%, followed by primary education at 26.7% and higher education at 25.5%. 87.6% of patients were residents of Commune VI.

2. The diaper mark

Among the 161 infants with diaper dermatitis, bulk thrift-store diapers were by far the most commonly used, with 74.52%, followed by non-bulk thrift-store diapers with 25.48%. There are few, if any, studies estimating the prevalence of bulk thrift store diaper use among infants in Mali.

In addition, the market is flooded with second-hand diapers, and their use with infants is really considerable due to their relatively low and accessible cost, with unit prices of 50, 75 or 100 FCFA.

3. Isolated mushrooms

Among the 161 infants, 24.85% of samples were collected and tested.

Of the samples tested, 47.5% were identified as *Candida albicans*, followed by *Candida lipolytica* (22.5%).

10% were identified as *Candida dubliniensis* and *Candida zeylanoides* respectively.

5% were identified for each of the species *Candida parapsilosis* and *Candida tropicalis.*

The *Revue Médicale de Liège 2006 has* practically the same tendency The most frequent complication of irritant diaper dermatitis is colonization of the injured skin by yeasts of the *Candida* genus. *Candida albicans* is most often involved, while others such as *Candida parapsilosis*, *Candida tropicalis*, *Candida. pulcherrina, Candida guillliermondii* and *Candida zeylanoides* are less common. This situation may correspond to diaper dermatitis colonized and aggravated by yeast, or to a true gluteal candidiasis infection [17].

4. Coat mark and isolated fungi

Of the *Candida albicans* isolated, 65% were in infants using bulk cloth diapers and 35% in those using non-bulk diapers.

100% of *Candida lipolytica* isolates were from infants using bulk cloth diapers.

Of the *Candida dubliniensis* isolated, 75% were in infants using bulk cloth diapers.

100% of *Candida zeylanoides* isolated were from infants using bulk cloth diapers.

Only one case of *Candida parapsilosis* candidiasis was associated with the Bulk Fripes diaper and the Non Fripes diaper respectively.

Similarly, one case of *Candida tropicalis* candidiasis was associated with the Bulk Fripes diaper and the Non Fripes diaper respectively.

The proportion of candidiasis in infants per diaper use differs significantly between Bulk Fripes and Non Fripes diapers ($p<0.01$) i.e. the percentage of candidiasis in infants per diaper use is greater when infants use Bulk Fripes diapers. .

However, given the relevant cosmopolitan and ubiquitous nature of the *Candida* genus, it is very difficult to strictly associate a species of the *Candida* genus with a specific brand of diaper. Other factors may also be taken into consideration, notably the conditions of manufacture, packaging, transport, storage, conservation and use of diapers in infants, which may also be limiting.

5. Limitations of our study:

5.1 Infant participation in the survey

Participation in the survey mainly concerned infants seen for diaper rash consultations in the pediatric department of Mali Hospital. For the infant's participation in the survey, the parents most often demand a full explanation, which seems normal, and we have not observed any case of refusal by the parents in relation to the infant's participation in the survey.

5.2 Image capture (photo) of candidiasis using diapers in infants

All the diaper rash images captured were on site at the Mali Hospital's pediatrics department. The reluctance of parents to capture images or take photos of diaper rash, even after a proposal and explanation of scientific, educational and total respect for anonymity, as well as the ethics and deontology of the profession, which demands respect for confidentiality. This reluctance is sometimes religious, cultural, linked to the parents' level of education, or simply a lack of confidence in the use of images.

5.3 Use of other products

The use of shea butter in place of preventive ointments such as oxyplastin prior to diaper use, the quality of the butter and its state of preservation. If shea butter is well preserved, its use on the diaper area avoids direct contact of the water contained in urine and feces with the skin, especially in the folds and convexities, thus considerably reducing diaper area moisture. Humidity and heat are the main factors favoring fungal infections, and if the butter is poorly preserved, it could be a factor in superinfection of the seat.

The use of traditional objects often made of rope, commonly called Tiélabagani in Bambara, which are too tight, causing irritation and can become superinfected and spread.

Reflex use of plant or plant derivative in traditional medicine for the treatment of diaper rash in infants.

Due to a lack of knowledge, the parents of infants self-medicate directly with antibiotics and/or corticosteroids instead of antifungals.

Powders are applied to diaper rash, sometimes at advanced stages in the infant's diaper area, out of total ignorance and with the intention of curing the condition.

The quality of the diaper is relevant through its synthetic or plastic nature, which has a tendency to promote heat production, maceration and even irritation not only of the infant's seat but also the waistband.

A good-quality diaper has a high proportion of absorbent materials, particularly cotton, with or without desiccant, and is the right size.

5.4 Sampling

The difficulties associated with sampling the infant's breech area are numerous, given the traditional treatments currently in use, notably the use of plants and shea butter, frequently used for both prevention and treatment. Modern medicines, especially antifungals, are used to treat oral candidiasis in infants. Ointments are also applied by self-medication, i.e. without a doctor's prescription, and aureomycin 3% is often used in this context. Powders used indiscriminately. Diaper rash is delimitable and tends to heal, which makes it difficult to remove it from the infant for routine mycological examination without further trauma. Cases of superinfection of the infant's diaper area due to the use of poorly preserved shea butter or other unsuitable products can be observed.

5.5 Limits to analysis performance

No use of selective or chromogenic media, making identification of the *Candida* genus easier and quicker.

CONCLUSION

Conclusion

We conducted a study of 161 infants with diaper dermatitis. These patients came exclusively from the pediatric ward of Hôpital du Mali. Tests to identify the *Candida* genus were carried out on site in the laboratory. 24.85% of samples were collected and tested.

55.28% were less than or equal to 6 months old (≤ 6 months), followed by the 6-12 months age group with 31.05%.

A sex ratio of 1.09

Bulk thrift store diapers, 74.52%, were by far the most popular.

Of the samples tested, 47.5% were identified as *Candida albicans.*

10% were identified as *Candida dubliniensis* and *Candida zeylanoides* respectively.

5% were identified as *Candida parapsilosis* and *Candida tropicalis* respectively.

Of the *Candida albicans* isolated, 65% were in infants using bulk cloth diapers.

100% of *Candida lipolytica* isolates were from infants using bulk cloth diapers.

Of the *Candida dubliniensis* isolated, 75% were in infants using bulk cloth diapers.

100% of *Candida zeylanoides* isolated were from infants using bulk cloth diapers.

The proportion of candidiasis in infants per diaper use was higher when infants used bulk fripe diapers. .

Performing genotyping tests and assessing the prevalence of the different *candida* species found in association with each other will improve our knowledge of candidiasis. The commitment of political authorities and communication to change behavior will help prevent candidiasis through the use of diapers in infants in Mali.

RECOMMENDATIONS

Recommendations

At the end of our study and in view of our results, we make the following recommendations:

To parents of newborn babies

- Pay special attention to currency exchange
- Personal hygiene
- Go to the nearest health facility

For clinicians

- Pay particular attention to the infant's breech during consultation
- Behavior Change Communication

Ministry of Health

- Make the means available (human, material and financial resources) for the prevention and management of mycological pathologies in general.
- Behavior Change Communication or Health Education

BIBLIOGRAPHICAL REFERENCES

References

1. R-V Talice. *Annales de Parasitologie Humaine et Comparée.* VIIIème edition (3-4), p. 394-410 . Paris : édition Masson ; 1930.
2. Professor Mouctar DIALLO. Les Candidoses [Cours]. Bamako: Institut National de Formation en Science de Santé; 2020.
3. GHASI, Asmaa. Diaper rash in infants and newborns: clinical manifestations and differential diagnosis [thesis]. RABAT: Université Mohammed V; 2016.
4. Haute Autorité de Santé France. Diaper rash [Internet]. HAS.2011. [cited December 7, 2011]. Available from: http://www.has-sante.frs
5. Boubacar Ahy Diatta, Rabak-Basba Mireille Nathalie Kabre,Salimatou Diallo Bèye, Fatimata Ly, Assane Kane, et al. Breech dermatitis in infants in Dakar: Study of 205 cases. 2017 ; 26(10) :1-4
6. Cynthia PIANETTI. Place of serodiagnosis in invasive fungal Candida infections. Survey on the prescription of Candida serologies at Nancy University Hospital and comparison of two commercial ELISA kits for the detection of mannan antigens and anti-mannan antibodies [thesis]. University of LORRAINE 2015.
7. Ms. BELAHCEN EL OUALI RITA. oral candidiasis in children [thesis]. RABAT: Université Mohammed V; 2016.
8. Frédéric Born. oral candidiasis: a review of the literature [thesis]. Geneva: University of Geneva; 2013
9. G-N Erasala, I Merlay, C Romain. *Archives de pédiatrie 14(5)*, p. 495-500 : Evolution des couches à usage unique et amélioration de l'état cutané du siège enfants . Paris : édition Masson ; Elsevier Masson SAS 2007.
10. L FERTITTA. Diaper rash. **réalités** Pédiatriques. Octobre 2019 ; n°234 : p.27-34 : Service de Dermatologie, Hôpital Necker-Enfants malades, PARIS.
11. Association Française des Enseignants de Parasitologie et Mycologie. Les Candidoses [Course]. UMVF - Université Médicale Virtuelle Francophone : (ANOFEL) 2014.
12. Manuel ANSEL and Cécile GAUTHIER. *Annales de Parasitologie Humaine et Comparée.* XXIXème edition (1-2), pp. 148-162. Paris : édition Masson ; 1954.
13. Dominique Tennstedt, Valérie Dekeuleneer. Contact dermatitis of the buttocks in infants and young children: is there only irritation. *Louvain médicale 137, 2018*; Dermatology Department, Cliniques Universitaires Saint-Luc, Brussels-Belgium.

14. Janis Crawford, Seydou Kane, Isabelle Lagarde, Patricia Raynault-Desgagné. Etude d'une solution alternative à l'utilisation de couches jetables en garderie [Diplôme supérieur en gestion de l'environnement]. Longueuil, Quebec, Canada: Université de Sherbrooke; April 22, 2006.
15. MALGRAIN Sandra. Dermatologie courante du nourrisson et du jeune enfant [Thesis]. ANGERS: Université Angers; October 28, 2014.
16. Béatrice GUERRIER. Les pathologies courantes chez les 0-2 ans: conseils à l'officine [thesis]. NANTES : Université de Nantes ; 2015.
17. Frédérique Henry, Laurence Thirion, Claudine Franchimont, Caroline Letawe, Gérald Pierard. *Revue Médicale de Liège 61 (4), 212-6, 2006*

APPENDIX

FACT SHEET

Name: KONATE

First name: Cheickna

Tel: + (223) 63 24 90 89 / 70 38 61 96 Email: cheicknako90@outlook.fr

Dissertation title: Diaper-related candidiasis in infants

Nationality: Malian

Academic year: 2019-2020

City of defense: Bamako/Mali

Place of delivery :

Areas of interest: Public health, Infectious diseases, Epidemiology, Mycology.

SUMMARY

Candidiasis is a cosmopolitan disease caused by ubiquitous ***Candida*** yeasts.

Irritant dermatitis or convex dermatitis is an erythematous dermatitis that starts at the areas where diapers rub, reaching the buttocks, external genitalia and thighs, forming a W shape and respecting the folds. Yeasts present in the stool can cause superinfection. In infants, diaper rash can develop very rapidly, particularly in the event of diarrhea.

Our study was conducted at Mali Hospital. It was a 10-month prospective descriptive study from July 2020 to April 2021. All infants with diaper dermatitis were included in our study. Species identification tests of the *Candida* genus were performed using the AUXACOLOR™2 gallery, the principle of which is based on the assimilation of sugars.

We conducted a study of 161 infants with diaper dermatitis. These patients came exclusively from the pediatric ward of Hôpital du Mali. Tests to identify the *Candida* genus were carried out on site in the laboratory. 24.85% of samples were collected and tested. 55.28% were aged less than or equal to 6 months (≤ 6 months), followed by the 6-12 months age group with 31.05%. A sex ratio of 1.09

Bulk thrift store diapers, 74.52%, were by far the most popular.

Of the samples tested, 47.5% were identified as *Candida albicans;* 10% as *Candida dubliniensis* and *Candida zeylanoides; and* 5% as *Candida parapsilosis* and *Candida tropicalis.*

Of the *Candida albicans* isolated, 65% were from infants using bulk cloth diapers; 100% of the *Candida lipolytica* isolated were from infants using bulk cloth diapers; Of the *Candida dubliniensis* isolated, 75% were from infants using bulk cloth diapers; 100% of the *Candida zeylanoides* isolated were from infants using bulk cloth diapers.

The proportion of candidiasis in infants per diaper use was higher when infants used bulk fripe diapers.

SURVEY FORM

STUDIES OF CANDIDIASIS IN INFANTS USING DIAPERS

Hôpital du Mali /service de pédiatrie, Bamako le 2020

Name:..

First names:...

Age :..Tel :..

Sex: F /____ / ; M /____/

Place of residence :

Commune I/____/ ; Commune II/____/ ; Commune III /____/ ; Commune IV /____/

Commune V/____/ ; Commune VI/____/ ; Others to be specified /____/ ....

Mother's **occupation**

Shopkeeper /____/ ; Pupil /____/ ; Student /____/ ; Housekeeper/____/

Household /____/ ; Others to be specified /____/ ....

Mother's level of education ;

Primary /____/ ; Secondary /____/ ; Higher education /____/ ; Others to be specified/____/................

Mother's marital status

1ère Epouse /____/ ; 2ème Epouse /____/ ; 3ème Epouse /____/ ; 4ème Epouse /____/

Clinical signs

Diaper rash/____/ ; Others to be specified/____/...

Isolated mushrooms

Candida. albicans /____/ ; Others to be specified /____/..

Diaper marks in infants

Fripe en Vrac /____/; Sweet baby® /____/; Sewa /____/; mamia® /____/; HiPP® /____/; Proprete® MINI /____/; Premaman MINI /____/; Libero *PEAUDOUCE* /____/; Baby dream® /____/; Lupilu®soft dry /____/; Hubbaby® /____/; Bien-Bien®/____/; LaLa bébé® /____/; CoCo bear®/____/ ; Panpanle®/____/ ; Baby Bliss®/____/ ; Happiesbaby®/____/ ; Other to be specified /____/..

IDENTIDICATION SHEET

Last Name: KONATE

First name: Cheickna

Tel: + (223) 63 24 90 89 / 70 38 61 96 Email: cheicknako90@outlook.fr

Title of the thesis: Candidiasis in infants by the use of diapers

Nationality: Malian

Academic year: 2019-2020

City of defense of thesis: Bamako / Mali

Place of deposit:

Focus Area: Public health, Infectious diseases, Epidemiology, Mycology.

SUMMARY

Candidiasis or moniliases are cosmopolitan conditions due to yeasts of the genus Candida ubiquitous.

Irritative dermatitis or convexities is an erythematous dermatitis starting at the areas of friction of the layer, reaching the buttocks, external genitalia, thighs, drawing a W and respecting the folds. Yeasts in the stool can cause superinfection. In infants, diaper rash can develop very quickly, especially in cases of diarrhea.

Our study was carried out at the Mali Hospital. This is a 10-month descriptive prospective study from July 2020 to April 2021. Any infant with brealymatitis by diaper use was included in our study. The species identification tests of the genus Candida were carried out by the AUXACOLOR gallery™2 whose principle is based on the assimilation of sugars.

We conducted a study of 161 infants with diaper dermatitis. These patients came exclusively from the pediatric ward of the Mali Hospital. Tests for identification of the Candida genus were performed on site in the laboratory department.

24.85% of samples were collected and tested.

55, 28% were less than or equal to 6 months old (≤ 6 months) followed by the 6-12 month age group with 31.05%. A sex ratio of 1,09

Bulk thrift store diapers, 74.52% were by far the most used.

Of the samples tested, 47.5% were identified as *Candida albicans*.

10% were identified as *Candida dubliniensis* and *Candida zeylanoides* respectively.

5% were identified as *Candida parapsilosis* and *Candida tropicalis* respectively.

Of the *Candida albicans* isolated, 65% were from infants using loose cloth diapers.

100% of *Candida lipolytica* isolated were from infants using bulk cloth diapers.

Of the *Candida dubliniensis* isolated, 75% were from infants using loose cloth diapers.

100% of *Candida zeylanoides* isolated were from infants using bulk cloth diapers.

The proportion of candidiasis in infants per diaper use was higher when infants used loose thrift diapers.

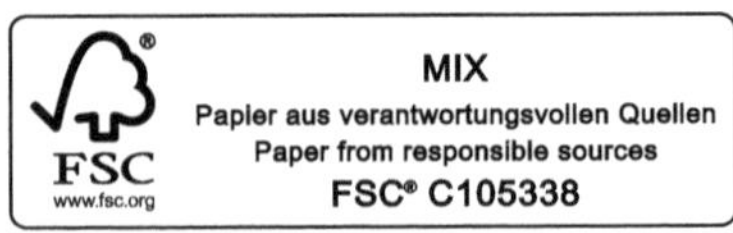

Printed by Books on Demand GmbH, Norderstedt / Germany